SHEDDING THE POUNDS

A COMPLETE SIMPLE
COOKBOOK FOR WOMEN

Dr Elizabeth J. Birdsong

TABLE OF CONTENT

INTRODUCTION

It doesn't matter if you're trying to lose weight or not;
everyone needs to eat well. Nonetheless, on the off chance
that weight reduction is your objective, good dieting turns out
to be much more significant. A well-balanced, nutrient-dense
diet not only helps you control how many calories you
consume, but it also gives your body the vitamins, minerals,
and other
nutrients it needs to work properly. A healthy diet helps people
lose weight, improve their overall health, and lower their risk of
chronic diseases like cancer, diabetes, and heart disease. Along
these lines, good dieting is a fundamental part of a fruitful get-
healthy plan.

BREAKFAST RECIPES FOR WEIGHT LOSS

Smoothie bowls

Smoothie bowls are a popular breakfast option that are not only delicious but also loaded with nutrients. Breakfast recipes for weight loss Smoothie bowls They are made by mixing healthy ingredients like fruits, vegetables, and nuts with other toppings like fresh fruit, seeds, and nuts. A basic smoothie bowl recipe and some nutritional information are provided here:

Ingredients:

1 cup of frozen natural product (like berries, mango, or pineapple)

1/2 cup of plain Greek yogurt

1/2 cup of unsweetened almond milk (or some other milk of your decision)

1/2 cup of spinach or kale leaves

1 tablespoon of honey or maple syrup (discretionary)

Blend the frozen fruit, Greek yogurt, almond milk, and leaves of spinach or kale in a blender.

Mix until smooth and rich.

In a bowl, pour the smoothie in.

Sliced banana, chopped nuts, or granola sprinkles are some of your favorite toppings.

Information on Nutrition: One serving of this recipe yields approximately:

Smoothie bowls contain between 250 and 300 calories, 15 to 20 grams of protein, 6 to 8 grams of fiber, 25 to 30 grams of carbohydrates, and 10 to 12 grams of fat. You can explore different avenues regarding various foods grown from the ground to make different flavors and surfaces. Simply make sure to pick sound fixings and watch segment sizes to guarantee that you stay inside your everyday calorie and supplement objectives.

Avocado toast is a popular breakfast or snack that is easy to make and tastes great. It's a simple dish with few ingredients that tastes good and is nutritious. An easy way to make avocado toast is as follows:

Ingredients:

1 ready avocado

2 cuts of bread (entire wheat or sourdough)

1 clove of garlic

1/2 lemon

Salt and pepper

Discretionary garnishes: tomato slices, feta cheese, a poached egg, smoked salmon, and other things

Instructions:

Toast the bread cuts in a toaster oven or on a frying pan until they are brilliant brown and fresh.

Cut the avocado in half lengthwise and remove the pit while the bread is toasting. Scoop the sort through of the avocado with a spoon and spot it in a little bowl.

Pound the avocado with a fork until it is smooth yet marginally stout. Mix the avocado well with the juice of half a lemon.

Strip the garlic clove and cut off the end. To impart garlic flavor, rub the cut end of the garlic clove over the surface of the toasted bread slices.

The garlic toast should be topped with the mashed avocado. To taste, sprinkle with salt and pepper.

Add any extra fixings you like, like cut tomatoes, feta cheddar, or a poached egg. Serve right away.

Healthy benefit: Avocado toast is a filling, healthy meal that has a good balance of protein, carbohydrates, and healthy fats. Using whole wheat bread and no additional toppings, one serving of avocado toast has the approximate following nutritional value:

Calories: 320 Fat: 18 grams of fat: 1.5 mg of cholesterol: Sodium: 0 mg: 260 milligrams of carbs: 35g Fiber: 11.5% Sugar: 3.5% protein: 10g

Nutritional value: Avocado is a decent wellspring of sound monounsaturated fats, which can assist with bringing down cholesterol and decrease the gamble of coronary illness. It is likewise plentiful in fiber, nutrients, and minerals, including vitamin E, vitamin K, folate, and potassium. Entire wheat bread gives complex starches and fiber, while garlic adds flavor and may have safe helping properties. In general, avocado toast is a filling and satisfying way to start your day.

Egg White Omelet with Veggies

Egg white omelets are a sound and protein-stuffed breakfast choice. They are simple to prepare and can be modified by adding your preferred vegetables and seasonings. An easy way to make an omelet with vegetables and egg whites is as follows:

Ingredients:

Three egg whites, one-quarter cup chopped vegetables (such as spinach, bell peppers, onions, and mushrooms), one teaspoon olive oil, and salt and pepper to taste

In a nonstick pan, heat the olive oil to a medium temperature.

Add the cleaved veggies and sauté until they are delicate, around 3-4 minutes.

In a little bowl, whisk the egg whites until they are foamy.

The egg whites should be poured into the pan and cooked for two to three minutes, or until the edges are set and the bottom has a light browned appearance.

Fold the omelet in half with a spatula and cook for an additional minute, or until the egg whites are cooked through.

Add salt and pepper to taste to the omelet before placing it on a serving plate. Serve right away.

Dietary benefit: Egg white omelets with veggies are a nutritious and low-calorie breakfast choice. Here is the rough dietary benefit of one serving:

Calories: 100 Fat: 2g Soaked fat: 0g Cholesterol: 0mg Sodium: 200mg Starches: 4g of fiber: 1g of sugar: 2g of protein: 16 grams of egg whites are a good source of protein and low in fat and cholesterol. Additionally, they are high in essential amino acids, which aid in muscle tissue development and repair. Veggies like spinach, ringer peppers, onions, and mushrooms are plentiful in nutrients, minerals, and cell reinforcements, which can assist with helping resistance and advance generally wellbeing. By utilizing olive oil rather than spread, you can lessen the soaked fat substance of this dish. In general, vegetable egg white omelets are a delicious and healthy way to start your day.

Greek Yogurt Parfait

Greek yogurt parfait is a sound and heavenly breakfast or tidbit that is not difficult to make and can be modified with your number one products of the soil. A straightforward recipe for Greek yogurt parfaits can be found here:

Ingredients:

1 cup Greek yogurt, 1/2 cup fresh berries (strawberries, blueberries, and raspberries, for example), 1/4 cup granola, and 1 tablespoon honey (optional)

Wash the berries and chop them into small pieces.

Blend the honey, if using, and Greek yogurt in a small bowl until smooth.

Layer the Greek yogurt, berries, and granola in alternating layers in a tall glass.

Keep layering until the glass is full, finishing with a layer of granola on top.

Cover and refrigerate until ready to serve, or serve immediately.

Nutrient density: A well-balanced breakfast or snack with a lot of protein, fiber, and essential vitamins and minerals is a Greek yogurt parfait. The approximate nutritional value of a single serving is as follows:

Calories: 350 Fat: 10g Immersed fat: 1 mg of cholesterol: Sodium: 0 mg: 100 milligrams of carbs: 43g Fiber: 7g of sugar: 20g Protein: Greek yogurt, which weighs 23 grams, is a good source of calcium and protein, both of which can aid in the development and upkeep of strong bones and muscles. Probiotics, which can help improve digestion and boost immunity, are also present in it, making it low in fat. Berries that are just picked have a lot of fiber, antioxidants, and vitamins C and K, all of which can help prevent and improve overall health. Granola contains complex carbohydrates and fiber, both of which can assist in controlling blood sugar levels and ensure that you feel full and satisfied. You can sweeten without adding refined sugar by using honey as a sweetener. In general, a healthy and delicious way to start the day or satisfy your sweet tooth is a Greek yogurt parfait.

Lunch Recipes for Weight Loss

Salad with Grilled Chicken: Weight Loss Lunch Recipes A salad with grilled chicken is a nutritious and delicious lunchtime dish. It is loaded with protein, fiber, and fundament

nutrients and minerals. A straightforward recipe for grilled chicken salad is provided here:

Ingredients:

2 cups mixed greens (such as lettuce, spinach, and arugula) 4 ounces grilled chicken breast, sliced 1/2 cup cherry tomatoes, halved 1/4 cup cucumber, sliced 1/4 cup red onion, and crumbled feta cheese Instructions:

Place the chopped mixed greens in a large salad bowl after being washed.

Top the greens with the cut barbecued chicken, cherry tomatoes, cucumber, and red onion.

Sprinkle the disintegrated feta cheddar over the top.

Toss the salad with the balsamic vinaigrette dressing to combine.

Close and keep in a fridge until ready to serve.

nutrient density: A well-balanced meal of salad and grilled chicken is full of protein, dietary fiber, and essential vitamins and minerals. The approximate nutritional value of a single serving is as follows:

Calories: 350 Fat: 18 grams of fat: 5g Cholesterol: Sodium: 85 mg: 700mg Carbs: 12g Fiber: 3.5% Sugar: 6g Protein: 35g

Barbecued chicken is a rich wellspring of protein and contains fundamental amino acids that assist fabricate and fix with muscling tissue. Mixed greens are low in calories and full of vitamins, minerals, fiber, and other nutrients that can help control digestion and improve overall health. Antioxidants and vitamins A and C are abundant in cherry tomatoes, which can boost immunity and protect against chronic diseases. Cucumber has a lot of water and few calories, which can help you stay hydrated and keep your skin healthy. Red onion is full of antioxidants and contains substances that can lower cholesterol and blood pressure. Feta cheese contains calcium and protein, but due to its high sodium content, it should be consumed in moderation. Served with your favorite vegetables and dressings, a salad with grilled chicken is a healthy and filling meal.

Veggie Wrap with Hummus

Veggie Wrap with Hummus A nutritious and flavorful veggie wrap with hummus is a quick and easy option for lunch or dinner. It's a great way to get a serving of vegetables and protein from plants. Here is a basic recipe for making a veggie wrap with hummus:

Ingredients:

Instructions: One large whole wheat wrap, 2 tablespoons hummus, 1/2 cup mixed vegetables (such as lettuce, bell peppers, and carrots), and 2 tablespoons crumbled feta cheese (optional).

Lay the entire wheat wrap on a spotless work surface.

Leave about one inch of space around the wrap's edges when spreading the hummus out evenly.

Organize the blended veggies over the hummus in an even layer.

If using, sprinkle the crumbled feta cheese on top.

Roll the wrap tightly after folding the edges in toward the center.

Slice the wrap down the middle and serve right away or envelop it with foil and take it with you in a hurry.

nutrient density: A well-balanced meal of vegetables wrapped in hummus is full of vitamins, minerals, and fiber. The approximate nutritional value of a single serving is as follows:

Calories: 300 Fat: 12g Immersed fat: 2 mg of cholesterol: Sodium, 5 mg: 600 milligrams of carbs: 35g of fiber: 7g of sugar: 6g Protein: A whole wheat wrap with 10 grams of fiber and complex carbohydrates can help you control your blood sugar and keep you full and satisfied. Healthy fats, which can assist in lowering cholesterol and reducing inflammation, can be found in hummus, which is a great source of plant-based protein. Fiber, vitamins, and minerals are abundant in mixed vegetables, which can aid in healthy digestion and overall health. Feta cheddar gives calcium and protein, yet it ought to be consumed with some
restraint because of its high sodium content. Generally, a veggie wrap with hummus is a solid and scrumptious method for getting in your day to day serving of veggies and supplements.

Turkey and Veggie Soup

Turkey and veggie soup is a warm and generous feast that is ideally suited for cooler climate. It is loaded with essential vitamins and minerals, protein, and fiber. A straightforward recipe for turkey and vegetable soup is as follows:

Ingredients:

1 lb ground turkey

1 onion, cleaved

2 garlic cloves, minced

2 carrots, cleaved

2 celery stems, cleaved

1 zucchini, cleaved

1 cup green beans, managed and cut into 1-inch pieces

1 can diced tomatoes (14 oz)

4 cups low-sodium chicken stock

2 tbsp olive oil

Salt and pepper, to taste

Guidelines:

With medium heat the Olive oil should be heated in a large dutch pot.

Add the ground turkey and cook until seared, around 5 minutes.

Cook for an additional two to three minutes, or until the onion is translucent, before adding the garlic.

Add the hacked carrots, celery, zucchini, and green beans to the pot and cook for 5-7 minutes, until the vegetables are marginally relaxed.

Season to taste with salt and pepper before adding the diced tomatoes and chicken broth.

After bringing the soup to a boil, reduce the heat to low and simmer for 20 to 30 minutes, or until the flavors have combined and the vegetables are tender.

If desired, top with shredded cheese or fresh herbs and serve hot.

nutrient density: A well-balanced meal of turkey and vegetable soup is full of protein, dietary fiber, and necessary vitamins and minerals. The approximate nutritional value of a single serving is as follows:

Calories: 240 Fat: 10g Immersed fat: 2 mg of cholesterol: Sodium, 50 mg: 700 milligrams of carbs: 16g Fiber: 5g Sugar: 8g Protein: 23g

Ground turkey is a lean protein source that is low in fat and calories, and it contains fundamental amino acids that assist fabricate and fix with muscling tissue. Carrots, celery, zucchini, and green beans are plentiful in fiber, nutrients, and minerals, which can assist with controlling assimilation and advance generally wellbeing. Vitamin C and lycopene, which can help prevent heart disease and cancer, can be found in diced tomatoes. Chicken stock adds flavor and gives electrolytes, which can assist with keeping up with legitimate hydration and control pulse. In general, turkey and vegetable soup is a nutritious and filling dish that can be enjoyed at any time of year.

Quinoa Salad with Roasted Vegetables

Quinoa salad with roasted vegetables is a light lunch or dinner option that is both healthy and delicious. It is loaded with essential vitamins and minerals, protein, and fiber. A straightforward recipe for quinoa salad with roasted vegetables is provided here:

Ingredients:

1 cup rinsed quinoa, 2 cups water, 2 cups chopped mixed vegetables (such as bell peppers, zucchini, eggplant, and cherry tomatoes), cut into bite-sized pieces, 2 tablespoons olive oil, 1 teaspoon dried thyme, salt and pepper to taste, 1/4 cup chopped fresh parsley, 1/4 cup chopped fresh mint, and 1/4 cup crumbled feta cheese (optional).

The oven should be heated to 400°F.

Bring the quinoa and water to a boil in a medium saucepan.

Decrease the intensity to low, cover the pot, and stew for 15-20 minutes, until the quinoa is delicate and the water has been assimilated.

In the mean time, spread the slashed vegetables in a solitary layer on a baking sheet.

Sprinkle the vegetables with thyme, salt, and pepper, and drizzle olive oil over them.

Toss the vegetables to evenly coat them, then roast for 20 to 25 minutes, or until they are tender and slightly charred.

In an enormous bowl, join the cooked quinoa, broiled vegetables, cleaved spices, and feta cheddar (if utilizing).

Shower the lemon juice and extra-virgin olive oil over the top, and throw to consolidate.

Quinoa salad should be served warm.

Dietary benefit: A well-balanced meal that is high in protein, dietary fiber, and essential vitamins and minerals is quinoa salad with roasted vegetables. The approximate nutritional value of a single serving is as follows:

Calories: 330 Fat: 17 grams of fat: 3 mg of cholesterol: Sodium, 8 mg: 160 milligrams of carbs: 37g of Fiber: 7g of sugar: 5g of protein: 10g

Quinoa is a finished protein source that contains each of the nine fundamental amino acids, as well as fiber, iron, and magnesium. Blended vegetables are plentiful in nutrients, minerals, and cell reinforcements, and can assist with helping resistance and safeguard against persistent sicknesses. Monounsaturated fats found in olive oil are beneficial for lowering cholesterol and inflammation. Herbs like mint and parsley enhance flavor and supply phytonutrients, which can assist in maintaining optimal health. Feta cheese contains calcium and protein, but due to its high sodium content, it should be consumed in moderation. In general, quinoa salad with broiled vegetables is a delightful and nutritious dinner that is not difficult to plan and ideal for any event.

DINNER RECIPES FOR WEIGHT LOSS

Grilled Fish with Roasted Vegetables

Barbecued fish with cooked vegetables is a solid and tasty dish that is not difficult to plan and ideal for a light and nutritious dinner. The ingredients and nutritional value of this easy recipe for grilled fish with roasted vegetables are listed below:

Ingredients:

4 fillets of your preferred fish, such as cod, tilapia, or salmon; 4 cups chopped mixed vegetables, such as bell peppers, zucchini, eggplant, and cherry tomatoes; 2 tablespoons olive oil; 1 teaspoon dried thyme; salt and pepper to taste; 1 lemon juice; 2 tablespoons chopped fresh parsley.

The oven should be heated to 400°F.

Spread the cleaved vegetables in a solitary layer on a baking sheet.

Shower the olive oil over the vegetables and sprinkle with thyme, salt, and pepper.

Throw to cover the vegetables equitably, and broil for 20-25 minutes, until the vegetables are delicate and somewhat burned.

Pre-heat a grill or grill pan to medium-high heat in the meantime.

Season the fish filets with salt, pepper, and lemon juice.

The fish fillets should be grilled for 3 to 4 minutes on each side, or until they are done.

Serve the barbecued fish with the simmered vegetables, and sprinkle with hacked parsley.

4 fillets of fish, 4 cups of mixed vegetables, 2 tablespoons olive oil, 1 teaspoon dried thyme, salt and pepper to taste, 1 lemon juice, 2 tablespoons chopped fresh parsley, and A well-balanced meal that is high in protein, dietary fiber, and essential vitamins and minerals is grilled fish with roasted vegetables. Here is the inexact dietary benefit of one serving:

Calories: 250 Fat: 12 grams of fat: 2g Cholesterol: Sodium, 60 mg: 120 milligrams of carbs: 10g Fiber: 4g of sugar: 5g of protein: 26g

Nutritional value: Fish is a rich wellspring of omega-3 unsaturated fats, which can assist with lessening irritation and lower the gamble of coronary illness. Vitamins, minerals, and antioxidants are abundant in mixed vegetables, which can help boost immunity and protect against chronic diseases. Monounsaturated fats found in olive oil are beneficial for lowering cholesterol and inflammation. Spices like thyme and parsley add flavor and give phytonutrients, which can assist with supporting ideal wellbeing. In general, barbecued fish with cooked vegetables is a tasty and nutritious dinner that is not difficult to plan and ideal for any event.

Baked Chicken with Sweet Potato Fries

Baked chicken with sweet potato fries is a satisfying and healthy dish that is simple to prepare. Baked chicken with sweet potato fries can be made in a few easy steps with the following ingredients and nutritional information:

Ingredients:

4 boneless, skinless chicken bosoms

2 huge yams, stripped and cut into fries

2 tbsp olive oil

1 tsp garlic powder

1 tsp smoked paprika

Salt and pepper, to taste

2 tbsp slashed new parsley

Directions:

The oven should be heated to 400°F.

Chicken breasts should be placed in parchment-lined baking sheet.

Season the chicken breasts with salt, pepper, garlic powder, smoked paprika, and olive oil.

Throw the yam fries with olive oil, and season with salt and pepper.

Spread the yam fries in a solitary layer on one more baking sheet fixed with material paper.

Heat the chicken and yam fries for 25-30 minutes, until the chicken is cooked through and the yam fries are firm and brilliant brown.

Serve the prepared chicken with the yam fries, and sprinkle with cleaved parsley.

Quantity of components:

4 boneless, skinless chicken breasts, 2 large sweet potatoes, 2 tablespoons olive oil, 1 teaspoon each of garlic powder and smoked paprika, salt and pepper to taste, and 2 tablespoons each of chopped fresh parsley A well-balanced meal that is high in protein, dietary fiber, and essential vitamins and minerals is baked chicken with sweet potato fries. Here is the inexact dietary benefit of one serving:

Calories: 400 Fat: 12 grams of fat: 2g Cholesterol: Sodium, 100 mg: 200 milligrams of carbs: 35g of fiber: 6g Sugar: 8g Protein: 35 grams of chicken provide a substantial amount of protein, which can aid in muscle growth and repair. Vitamin A, fiber, and complex carbohydrates found in sweet potatoes can support healthy skin and eyes, digestion, and immunity. Monounsaturated fats found in olive oil are beneficial for lowering cholesterol and inflammation. Garlic and parsley are two examples of herbs that add flavor and contain phytonutrients that can support optimal health. In general, baked chicken with sweet potato fries is a filling, delicious, and simple dish that is appropriate for any occasion.

Stir-Fry Vegetables with Tofu

Stir-fry vegetables with tofu is a sound and delicious dish that is not difficult to make and ideal for a speedy and nutritious dinner. Tofu stir-fry vegetables can be made in a simple recipe with the following ingredients and nutritional information:

Ingredients:

1 block of firm tofu, depleted and cut into solid shapes

1 tbsp vegetable oil

1 tbsp soy sauce

1 tbsp cornstarch

1 onion, cut

2 chime peppers, cut

2 cups broccoli florets

2 cups cut mushrooms

2 cloves garlic, minced

1 tbsp ground ginger

Salt and pepper, to taste

Directions:

In a bowl, whisk together the vegetable oil, soy sauce, and cornstarch.

Toss in the tofu cubes to ensure an even coating. Place aside.

In a large skillet, heat the oil to medium-high.

Cook the marinated tofu on all sides in the skillet until it is golden brown. Eliminate from the skillet and put away.

Add the bell peppers and onion to the same skillet and cook for two to three minutes.

Add the broccoli, mushrooms, garlic, and ginger, and cook for an extra 5-7 minutes, or until the vegetables are delicate fresh.

Return the tofu to the skillet and throw with the vegetables.

Season with salt and pepper, to taste.

Quantity of components:

1 block firm tofu, 1 tablespoon vegetable oil, 1 tablespoon soy sauce, 1 tablespoon cornstarch, 1 onion, 2 bell peppers, 2 cups broccoli florets, 2 cups sliced mushrooms, 2 cloves of garlic, 1 tablespoon grated ginger, salt and pepper to taste Pan sear vegetables with tofu is a low-calorie, high-protein, and supplement thick feast that is loaded with fiber, nutrients, and minerals. Here is the inexact dietary benefit of one serving:

Calories: 250 Fat: 11 grams of fat: 1 mg of cholesterol: Sodium: 0 mg: 500mg Carbs: 23g of fiber: 6g Sugar: 8g Protein: 17 grams of tofu contain a lot of calcium and plant-based protein, both of which can support bone health and muscle function.

Nutritional value: Vegetables like broccoli, ringer peppers, and mushrooms are plentiful in cell reinforcements, fiber, and nutrients, which can assist with lessening irritation, help resistance, and backing ideal wellbeing. Soy sauce adds flavor and provides essential amino acids, while garlic and ginger offer immune-boosting and anti-inflammatory properties. In general, stir-fry vegetables with tofu are a delicious and nutritious dish that is simple to prepare and ideal for a diet that is both healthy and well-balanced.

Turkey Meatballs with Zucchini Noodles

Turkey meatballs with zucchini noodles are an excellent low-carb, high-protein dish that is both nutritious and filling. A straightforward recipe for turkey meatballs using zucchini noodles is provided, along with the quantities of the ingredients and their nutritional value:

Ingredients:

1 lb. ground turkey, 1/4 cup almond flour, 1 egg, 1 tbsp. olive oil, 1 tsp. garlic powder, 1 tsp. onion powder, salt and pepper to taste, 2 spiralized large zucchini, 1 jar of tomato sauce, and chopped fresh basil (optional).

Instructions

Preheat the stove to 375°F (190°C).

In a bowl, combine as one the ground turkey, almond flour, egg, olive oil, garlic powder, onion powder, salt, and pepper until very much joined.

Shape the blend into little meatballs, around 1 inch in breadth.

Meatballs should be kept on a parchment-lined baking sheet.

Bake the meatballs for 15 to 20 minutes, or until they are cooked through.

In a huge skillet, heat the pureed tomatoes over medium intensity.

Cook the zucchini noodles for five to seven minutes, or until they are soft.

If desired, top the zucchini noodles with turkey meatballs and fresh basil.

Quantity of components:

1 lb. ground turkey, 1/4 cup almond flour, 1 egg, 1 tablespoon olive oil, 1 teaspoon garlic powder, 1 teaspoon onion powder, salt and pepper to taste, 2 large zucchini, 1 jar of tomato sauce, chopped fresh basil (optional) Turkey meatballs with zucchini noodles are a low-carb, high-protein dish loaded with antioxidants, vitamins, and minerals. Here is the inexact dietary benefit of one serving:

Calories: 350 Fat: 18 grams of fat: 4 mg of cholesterol: Sodium, 120 mg: 550mg Carbs: 18g of fiber: 5g of sugar: 10 g of protein: 29 grams of turkey is a low-saturated-fat, high-essential-amino acid protein source that can support muscle growth and repair.

Nutritional value: The meatballs benefit from the texture and flavor of almond flour, which is a gluten-free and low-carb alternative to breadcrumbs. Zucchini noodles are a low-calorie, low-carb option in contrast to customary pasta that are plentiful in fiber and nutrients, which can assist with advancing stomach related wellbeing and resistance. Pureed tomatoes is a decent wellspring of lycopene, a strong cell reinforcement that can help safeguard against oxidative pressure and ongoing sicknesses. Fresh basil adds flavor and has antibacterial and anti-inflammatory properties. In general, turkey meatballs with zucchini noodles is a heavenly and nutritious dinner that is not difficult to make and ideal for a solid and adjusted diet.

SNACKS AND DESSERTS FOR WEIGHT LOSS

37

Fruit Salad with Yogurt

Fruit salad with yogurt is a delicious and healthy snack or dessert that is easy to make and perfect for any occasion. Here's a simple recipe for making fruit salad with yogurt along with the nutritional value of the dish.

Ingredients:

2 cups of plain Greek yogurt

2 cups of mixed fresh fruit (such as strawberries, blueberries, grapes, kiwi, mango, pineapple, and/or oranges)

1 tablespoon of honey

1 teaspoon of vanilla extract

The should be washed first and chopped into bite-sized.

In a large bowl, mix the Greek yogurt, honey, and vanilla extract until well combined.

Add the fruit to the bowl and gently mix until the fruit is coated with the yogurt mixture.

It can be kept in the fridge or taken immediately.

Nutritional value:

This fruit salad with yogurt is packed with essential nutrients and vitamins. Here's the nutritional value of one serving (based on 2 cups of mixed fruit and 2 cups of Greek yogurt):

Calories: 400

Protein: 34g

Fat: 5g

Carbohydrates: 61g

Fiber: 8g

Sugar: 48g

Sodium: 160mg

Calcium: 40% DV

Vitamin C: 160% DV

Iron: 6% DV

This fruit salad with yogurt is high in protein and low in fat, making it a healthy and filling snack or dessert. The mixed fruit provides a variety of vitamins and minerals, such as vitamin C, fiber, and potassium. The Greek yogurt is a great source of calcium, which is important for maintaining strong bones and teeth. The honey adds a touch of sweetness, but you can adjust the amount of honey to your taste preference. Enjoy this delicious and nutritious fruit salad with yogurt anytime of the day!

Kale chips

Kale chips are a healthy and delicious snack that can be easily made at home. Here is a simple recipe for making kale chips along with the nutritional value of the dish.

Ingredients:

1 bunch of kale

1 tablespoon of olive oil

1/2 teaspoon of salt

Instructions:

Preheat your oven to 350°F (175°C).

Wash the kale and remove the stems. Tear the leaves into bite-sized pieces.

Place the kale pieces in a large bowl and drizzle with olive oil. Use your hands to massage the oil into the leaves.

Sprinkle with salt and toss to coat.

Place the kale pieces in a single layer on a baking sheet lined with parchment paper.

Bake for 10-15 minutes, or until the kale is crispy and slightly browned.

It should be removed from the oven and allowed to cool for some time then served.

Nutritional values

Kale chips are good substitutes to potato chips. Here's the nutritional value of one serving of kale chips (based on one bunch of kale, one tablespoon of olive oil, and 1/2 teaspoon of salt):

Calories: 150

Protein: 7g

Fat: 11g

Carbohydrates: 12g

Fiber: 4g

Sugar: 1g

Sodium: 600mg

Vitamin A: 590% DV

Vitamin C: 320% DV

Calcium: 25% DV

Iron: 20% DV

Kale is a superfood that is rich in vitamins and minerals, especially vitamin A and vitamin C. It is also high in fiber and low in calories, making it a great choice for snacking. The olive oil provides healthy fats that are good for the heart, and the salt adds flavor. However, it's important to note that kale chips are high in sodium, so if you are on a low-sodium diet, you may want to reduce the amount of salt used in this recipe. Enjoy these delicious and healthy kale chips as a snack anytime of the day!

Dark Chocolate Almonds

Dark chocolate almonds are a tasty and healthy snack that can be easily made at home. Here is a simple recipe for making dark chocolate almonds along with the nutritional value of the dish.

Ingredients:

1 cup of raw almonds

1/2 cup of dark chocolate chips

1   tablespoon   of   coconut   oil

1/4 teaspoon of sea salt

:

Preheat your oven to 350°F (175°C).

Spread the almonds in a single layer on a baking sheet and toast in the oven for 10-15 minutes, or until lightly browned and fragrant.

In a double boiler or a heatproof bowl set over a pot of simmering water, melt the dark chocolate chips and coconut oil, stirring occasionally.

Once the chocolate is melted, remove from heat and add the toasted almonds to the bowl. Stir until the almonds are coated with the chocolate mixture.

The chocolate-covered almonds should be spread in a single layer on a parchment-lined baking sheet.

Sprinkle with sea salt and let cool at room temperature until the chocolate has hardened.

Once the chocolate has hardened, break the almonds apart and serve.

Dark chocolate almonds are a healthy snack that combines the benefits of dark chocolate and almonds. Here's the nutritional value of one serving of dark chocolate almonds (based on 1 cup of raw almonds, 1/2 cup of dark chocolate chips, 1 tablespoon of coconut oil, and 1/4 teaspoon of sea salt):

Calories: 450

Protein: 11g

Fat: 35g

Carbohydrates: 33g

Fiber: 10g

Sugar: 17g

Sodium: 150mg

Iron: 25% DV

Magnesium: 25% DV

Potassium: 10% DV

Almonds are a great source of protein and healthy fats, while dark chocolate is high in antioxidants and may have benefits for heart health. The addition of sea salt adds a touch of flavor, but be mindful of the amount of salt used if you are on a low-sodium diet. Enjoy these delicious and nutritious dark chocolate almonds as a snack anytime of the day!

45

Peanut Butter Energy Balls

Peanut butter energy balls are a quick and easy snack that's perfect for when you need a quick boost of energy. Here is a simple recipe for making peanut butter energy balls along with the nutritional value of the dish.

Ingredients:

1 cup of rolled oats

1/2 cup of natural peanut butter

1/4 cup of honey

1/4 cup of mini chocolate chips

1/4 cup of ground flaxseed

1/4 cup of shredded coconut

1 teaspoon of vanilla extract

Instructions:

In a large mixing bowl, combine the rolled oats, peanut butter, honey, mini chocolate chips, ground flaxseed, shredded coconut, and vanilla extract. Stir until well combined.

Cover the bowl with plastic wrap and chill in the refrigerator for at least 30 minutes, or until the mixture is firm enough to roll into balls.

Using a tablespoon or a small cookie scoop, portion the mixture into balls and roll between your palms until smooth.

Place the peanut butter energy balls on a baking sheet lined with parchment paper.

Chill the peanut butter energy balls in the refrigerator for at least 1 hour, or until firm.

Once firm, the energy balls can be stored in an airtight container in the refrigerator for up to 2 weeks.

Nutritional value:

Peanut butter energy balls are a nutritious snack that's packed with protein and fiber. Here's the nutritional value of one serving of peanut butter energy balls (based on 1 cup of rolled oats, 1/2 cup of natural peanut butter, 1/4 cup of honey, 1/4 cup of mini chocolate chips, 1/4 cup of ground flaxseed, 1/4 cup of

shredded coconut, and 1 teaspoon of vanilla extract,
yielding approximately 16 energy balls):

Calories: 140

Protein: 4g

Fat: 8g

Carbohydrates: 15g

Fiber: 2g

Sugar: 9g

Sodium: 40mg

Peanut butter is a good source of protein and healthy fats,
while oats, ground flaxseed, and shredded coconut
provide fiber and other nutrients. Honey and mini
chocolate chips add sweetness and flavor, but be mindful
of the amount of sugar used if you are on a low-sugar diet.
These peanut butter energy balls are a convenient and
healthy snack that can help keep you fueled throughout
the day.

MEAL PLANNING AND PREP TIPS

48

Eating healthy and losing weight requires discipline and planning, but having the right kitchen essentials can make it easier. Here are some kitchen essentials that can help you eat healthy and achieve your weight loss goals.

Food scale A food scale can help you accurately measure portion sizes, which is essential for managing your calorie intake.

Non-stick cookware Non-stick cookware can help you cook with less oil and fat, which can help reduce your calorie intake. It also makes cleaning up easier.

Steamer basket A steamer basket can help you cook vegetables without adding oil or fat. Steamed vegetables are a great addition to any healthy meal.

.

Blender A blender can help you make smoothies and soups that are packed with nutrients. It's also great for making homemade sauces and dressings.

Air fryer An air fryer can help you cook foods with less oil, making them healthier and lower in calories. It's also great for cooking crispy vegetables and chicken.

Quality knives Investing in quality knives can make meal prep easier and safer. A sharp knife can help you quickly chop vegetables and fruits without risking injury.

Food storage containers Having a variety of food storage containers can help you portion out your meals and snacks. This help you prevent overeating.

Measuring cups and spoons Measuring cups and
spoons can help you accurately measure out ingredients
for recipes. It helps you in monitoring your calorie intake
and prevents overeating.

By having these kitchen essentials on hand, you can make
healthy eating and weight loss easier and more
convenient. With a little planning and preparation, you
can achieve your weight loss goals and enjoy delicious,
nutritious meals.

Healthy Substitutions for High-Calorie Ingredients

Making healthy substitutions for high-calorie
ingredients is a great way to reduce
your calorie intake without sacrificing flavor. Here are
some healthy substitutions you can try in your cooking and
baking:

Greek yogurt instead of sour cream Greek yogurt is a
great substitute for sour cream in recipes. It has a similar
texture and tangy flavor, but is lower in calories and
higher in protein.

Spaghetti squash instead of pasta Spaghetti squash is a
great low-carb alternative to

pasta. It has a similar texture and can be used in place of spaghetti noodles in recipes.

Almond flour instead of all-purpose flour Almond flour is a great gluten-free alternative to all-purpose flour. It has less carbs and contains more in protein and healthy fats.

Cauliflower rice instead of white rice Cauliflower rice is a great low-carb alternative to white rice. It has a similar texture and can be used in place of rice in recipes.

Avocado instead of mayonnaise Mashed avocado is a great substitute for mayonnaise in recipes. It has a similar creamy texture and is higher in healthy fats and nutrients.

Zucchini noodles instead of pasta Zucchini noodles, also known as zoodles, are a great low-carb alternative to pasta. They can be used in place of noodles in recipes.

Ground turkey instead of ground beef Ground turkey is a leaner alternative to ground beef. It is lower in calories and saturated fat, but still high in protein.

Applesauce instead of oil Applesauce is a great substitute for oil in baking recipes. It is
lower in calories and fat, but still helps keep baked goods moist.

By making these healthy substitutions, you can reduce your calorie intake and increase your nutrient intake without sacrificing flavor or satisfaction. Experiment with these substitutions in your favorite recipes and see how they can help you achieve your health goals.

Planning and preparing meals for the week can help you save time and money, reduce food waste, and make healthier choices. A simple weekly meal planner has been attached below to help organize better choice of food.

WEEKLY MEAL PLANNER

54

BREAKFAST LUNCH DINNER SNACK

MON

TUE

WED

THU

FRI

SAT

SUN

NAME:............,........................

WEEKLY MEAL PLANNER

55

BREAKFAST   LUNCH.   DINNER   SNACK

MON

TUE

WED

THU

FRI

SAT

SUN

NAME:......................................

WEEKLY MEAL PLANNER

56

BREAKFAST.   LUNCH.   DINNER   SNACK

MON

TUE

WED

THU

FRI

SAT

SUN

NAME:.................................

WEEKLY MEAL PLANNER

57

	BREAKFAST.	LUNCH	DINNER	SNACK
MON				
TUE				
WED				
THU				
FRI				
SAT				
SUN				

NAME:...

WEEKLY MEAL PLANNER

58

BREAKFAST   LUNCH   DINNER.   SNACK

MON

TUE

WED

THU

FRI

SAT

SUN

NAME:......................................

WEEKLY MEAL PLANNER

59

BREAKFAST.   LUNCH   DINNER   SNACK

MON

TUE

WED

THU

FRI

SAT

SUN

NAME:..

WEEKLY MEAL PLANNER

BREAKFAST   LUNCH   DINNER   SNACK

MON

TUE

WED

THU

FRI

SAT

SUN

NAME:..

WEEKLY MEAL PLANNER

61

	BREAKFAST	LUNCH	DINNER.	SNACK
MON				
TUE				
WED				
THU				
FRI				
SAT				
SUN				

NAME:...

WEEKLY MEAL PLANNER

	BREAKFAST	LUNCH	DINNER	SNACK
MON				
TUE				
WED				
THU				
FRI				
SAT				
SUN				

NAME:...

WEEKLY MEAL PLANNER

63

BREAKFAST　LUNCH　DINNER　SNACK

MON

TUE

WED

THU

FRI

SAT

SUN

NAME:.................................

WEEKLY MEAL PLANNER

64

	BREAKFAST	LUNCH	DINNER	SNACK
MON				
TUE				
WED				
THU				
FRI				
SAT				
SUN				

NAME:....,..............................

CONCLUSION

Healthy eating is a crucial aspect of weight loss for women. Women have unique nutritional needs that require a balanced and nutrient-dense diet to promote weight loss, improve overall health, and reduce the risk of chronic diseases. A healthy diet should include plenty of fruits, vegetables, whole grains, lean protein, and healthy fats while limiting processed foods, sugar, and saturated and trans fats. Additionally, it's essential to practice portion control, stay hydrated, and engage in regular physical activity. Adopting healthy eating habits can be challenging, but the benefits are well worth the effort. By making small changes to your diet and lifestyle, you can achieve your weight loss goals, feel better, and live a healthier, more fulfilling life.

Thank you...

www.ingramcontent.com/pod-product-compliance
Lightning Source LLC
Chambersburg PA
CBHW050053260726
48658CB00005B/1936